Copyright © 2019 by Calpine Composition Notebooks
All rights reserved. This book or any portion thereof
may not be reproduced or used in any manner whatsoever
without the express written permission of the publisher.

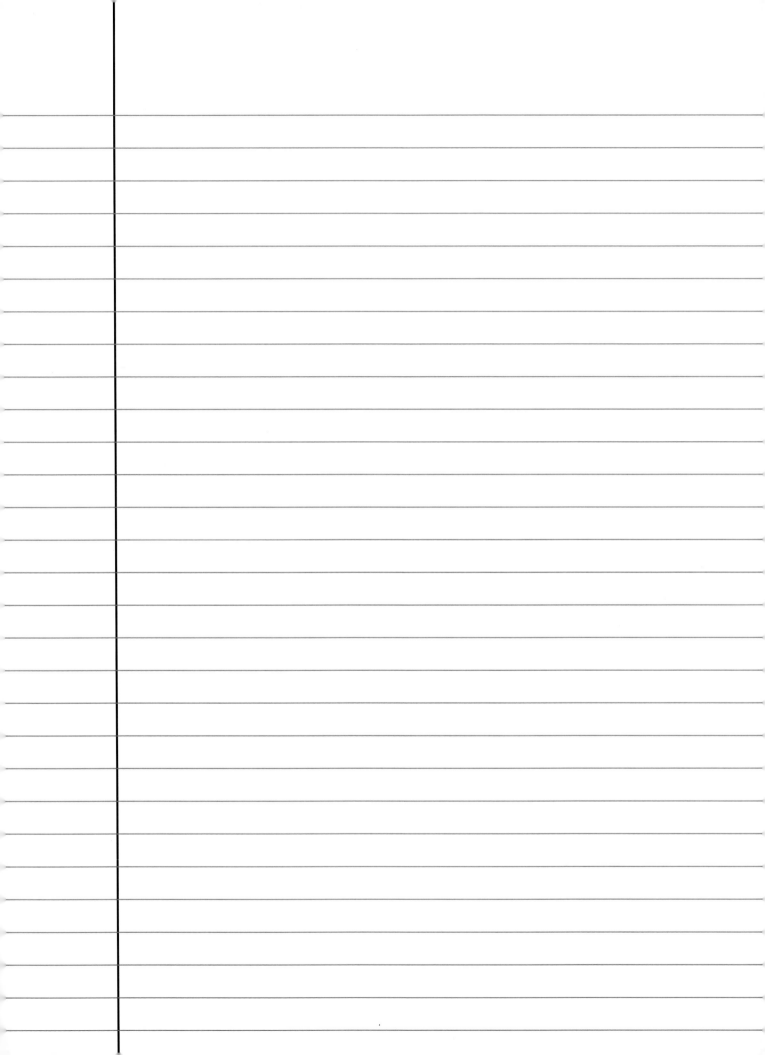

Made in United States
North Haven, CT
01 June 2022